HEALING BY QI
Published by Dzung Dang Van
Copyright 2018 Dzung Dang Van

Legal Notice

* When you pay for downloading the copies of this e-book, you can share with your family members to bring you practical benefits by practicing together. But that does not mean you have the right to share this e-book free on the Internet and social networking sites because this action means you have violated ethical issues and copyrights.

* The author and publisher of this E-book and the accompanying materials have used their best efforts in preparing this E-book. The author and publisher make no representation or warranties with respect to the accuracy, applicability, fitness, or completeness of the contents of this E-book. The information contained in this E-book is strictly for educational purposes. Therefore, if you wish to apply ideas contained in this E-book, you are taking full responsibility for your actions.

* The author and publisher disclaim any warranties (express or implied), merchantability, or fitness for any particular purpose. The author and publisher shall in no event be held liable to any party for any direct, indirect, punitive, special, incidental or other consequential damages arising directly or indirectly from any use of this material, which is provided "as is", and without warranties.

Contents

Chapter 1 - Overview

Chapter 2 - The division of yin and yang on the human body

Chapter 3 - The effect of the mind on the qi flow

Chapter 4 - The qi release by hand waving technique

Chapter 5 - The qi release technique to a point

Chapter 6 - The qi release by massaging techniques

Chapter 7 - The qi release by blowing techniques

Chapter 8 - The objects hold qi

Chapter 9 - Healing by qigong

Chapter 10 - Practice qigong to healing

Conclusions

Chapter 1

Overview

Many person don't know that people is an energy receiver machine and release - where does this capacity come from? We all have it from birth, like we have muscular force, but genetics affect its intensity. Energy in body also affects our health and body condition. Some people have this super energy because of congenital or after experiencing a deadly event. Others have the super energy due to practice the exercise. They may inadvertently cause an attractive, balanced, comforting, healing effect on those around them.

However, do not assume that the influence of heredity is impossible to attack and endure the disabilities when born until death or enjoy good health forever no matter what happens. Our energy is not fixed, but it can change drastically if we persist in following the rules of healthy living. If we do not work too hard or too little then our balance also helps our organs self-repair their daily wear and tear. If we manage the vibrations to save our nerve power, we will become rich in energy, nerve power and vigor.

The balance of the body, the autonomy, the rational development of the mental functions is the goals of those who wish to attain the qi full status. No one can conquer this capacity, if not carefully supervised body or forget that the apparatus in the body are reciprocal. If you want to maintain a perfect and long-lasting state of qi, take care of the three components: The body, consciousness and subconscious are balanced.

Some mentally weak or physically damaged but it makes us think they have a lot of energy. They are like being received the special gifts of universe, but actually their energy will be exhausted soon. Because the energy of the qi body closely connect to the physical and mental state.

So the persons wants to become a qi column, the first is that they must conquer health and self-control. Next, they have to consciously use their accumulation and storage capacities, but their mind should be strong, quiet, persistent, always calm and wise. The impulsive persons will let them be caught up in anger, the timid persons let themselves loose in temporary courage, all them are not heroes. Because when their excitement disappears, they fall back to motionlessness. To control others, we have to control our nerves. Before we think about giving out energy, we have to feel the full energy status in ourselves.

Addition, do not assume that the emission of qi by well-developed people makes them tired, wasting energy stored in their bodies. Oppose thing, this is an excellent exercise. Like an athlete who draws a lot of new power in his daily exercise, the qigong master grows stronger his energy. The release of qi to healing is opportunistic and the preserve energy is far from exhausted, it is constantly nourished. So the qigong master is not afraid to lose energy. The nerve tufts will continually recharge new energy to replenish losses. Of course, the first actions should not be too eager to foolish level. If you overdo it, you'll get aches: muscles that are clogged by dead cells will become stiff and painful. This is the same for the primary qigong who want to abuse their powers to mislead, without taking into account their weakness. However, this situation is not worrying, a few minutes of relaxation, a series of deep breaths of new strength. Normally, after re-loading the nerve center, the person is stronger than before, has a wonderful feeling of comfort, fitness, balance, physical and mental freedom.

Evidence of the harmlessness of qigong is that famous qigong masters lived for so long. The older masters cure the disease faster and more people.

The yang nerve tufts of the sympathetic nervous system pulsate as well as qi storage centers. This energy spreads the whole body, distributes according to certain rules and divides the yin and yang according to the region in which it expressed.

When not self-limiting in the human form, this energy forms around the body of an atmosphere, often called the "halo".

Let's do the following experiment: Place a magnet on a paper cover, on which a thin layer of iron is spread. Tap softly on the paper, you see the iron folds as shown below.

The iron particles are attracted by an invisible force that gathers in certain directions, particularly thicker at the poles.

The human body is subject to the same rules. At every times, people also emit energy as well as magnets which also have a positive electrode and negative electrode that create attraction and thrust.

If you have the well health and complete self-control by strong will, your aura will be broad and strong. You can control or regulate the release of this energy by the will to direct it to a certain part of the body.

The self-suggestion by concentrating thought can be put this energy into positive nerve tufts and from there to release in a certain direction.

Our gestures combined with the effect above make the release of qi easy and the eyes can also make more effective. Finally, some items like wax, water, cotton swabs can be charged and stored qi like light absorbers or electrical attractants. These are real qi convergence objects.

Chapter 2

The division of yin and yang on the human body

According to experimental works in the West, especially the baron Reichenbach, the

Austrian psychiatrist and Dr. Hector Dunville, humans are like two "horseshoe" magnets of different size which are put together. Large horseshoe magnet is represented the yin yang of two body sides, small horseshoe magnet is expressed yin yang of front and back. The two branches of the large magnet exhibit two arms and two legs, the right is positive (+) and the left is negative (-). The neutral point is at the top of the head. A small magnet is placed in the opposite position. The neutral point is at the bottom of the pelvis. The front branch which goes from the abdomen to the forehead is positive (+), the second branch which goes from the kidneys to the nape is the negative (-). There are few exceptions. If someone is left-handed then the left side is positive (+), right side is negative (-). The chest and back do not change. Just like electric power escapes from the spikes, the limbs are the main part to release the qi. The right hand releases the yang qi (+), the left hand releases the yin qi (-). Indian yogis have the same opinion.

When we put the two magnets together, the positive electrode face to the cathode and vice versa then two are attracted to each other. Conversely, when the two positive electrode or two cathode opposite each other then they will push each other. The human body also has the same phenomenon. Placing the right hand on the forehead will have the pushing force which a sensitive person can recognize. In contrast, putting your left hand on your forehead will have a suck force. Pushing force creates an effect of excitement, while the suck force creates a effect of reassuring, appeasing. Therefore, to relieve for the patient, we must put our right hand in front of the left chest and left hand in front the right chest of patients. When we want to excite them, we cross our hands.

In short, there are three rules:

1. The human body can be divided into yin and yang: The right is yang, the left is yin; the front is yang; the back is yin.

2. The yin and yang of the right and left sides can be reversed for left-handed people.

The yin and yang of the front and rear do not change.

3. Yang opposite yang or yin opposite yin is excitement. Yang opposite yin or yin opposite yang is a placating.

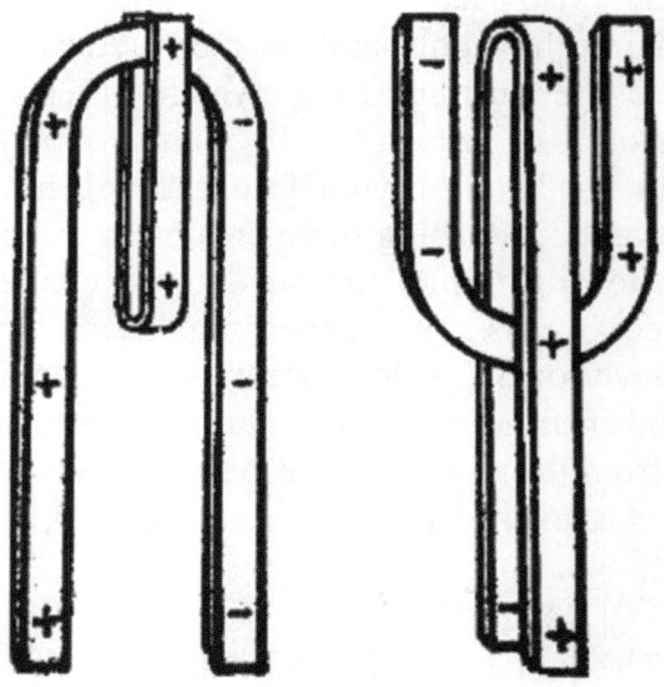

Figure 1- The icon of yin and yang divisions on the human body

Above is the yin and yang distribution on the human body at the general level. Actually the problem is much more complication, besides the general yin yang have yin-yang details. Take a look at the example of right hand: The above mentioned hand was positive (+); this is true because the yang dominates there, but inside there are traces of yin. The arms are divided into two parts along the long limb, the yin part on the side of the thumb and the yang part on the side of the little finger. It is the yin in yang and yang in the yang. Going further with each finger, the fingers which are near the thumb have a yin attribute and the fingers which are near the little finger have a yang attribute. The same to the foot, the part along the foot at side of the forefoot has a yin attribute, while the rest at side of the little toe has a yang attribute. The toes which are near forefoot have a yin attribute and the toes which are near the little-toe have a yang attribute. On the mouth, the upper lip is yang (+), while the lower lip is yin (-). At the general level, the yang factors (+) dominates at the male, the yin factors (-) predominates at the female.

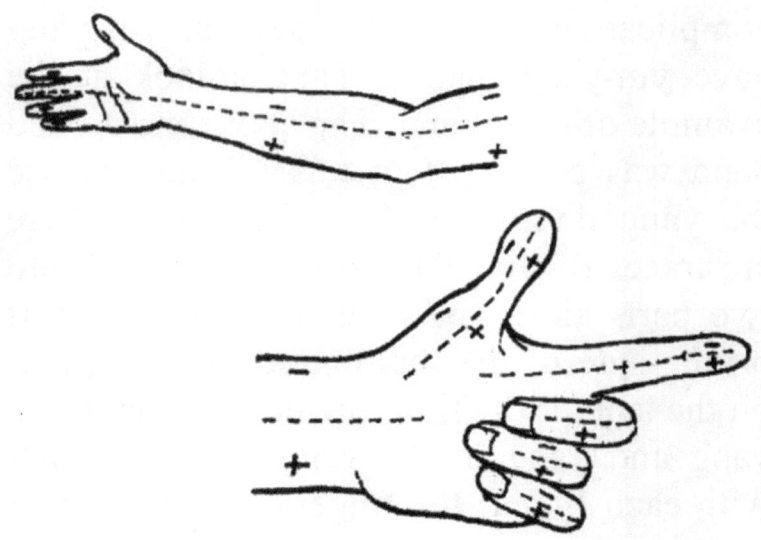

Figure 2 - The yin and yang divisions of a hand

Chapter 3

The effect of the mind on the qi flow

You can use the will to drive the qi arbitrarily. Your mind makes the qi to become harmonize, easy to control and many different characteristics. How do qi spread? It's in waveform. What happens if you throw rocks into the lake? The circles form, grow large, and weaker as the farther away. Keep a hot object near the side of a cold object. The heat radiates each wave into a cold object and transfers heat until a temperature equilibrium exists between the two objects. Everything is shining like that, but different intensity. Two people who have the different strong minds close together like hot objects near cold objects. Each person radiates a field of influence according to the strength of his mind. When two qi fields collide, they infiltrate each other until they reach equilibrium: The weaker who is under average will suck and the strength of the strong and add a new power to increase his vitality. Therefore, the qi gong master must be healthy, self-reliant, balanced as much as possible physically and mentally. Physicians who weaken the balance loss can only be transmitted to patients with his disease.

The mind influences the qi flow, communicating a particular vividness, a vibration of atoms constituting the body. Sometimes we lack the courage, strength, vitality then body's vibration is not enough to cure effective. On the contrary, when we angry or irritate overstimulation, the vibration of body is very strong. Only when our mind is in state of total quietness, we just get important results. Therefore, qi gong masters must increase their self-efficacy and place themselves in a state of physical and mental similarity to the state they wish to achieve in the patient. For helping patient relieving their negativity the doctor must ready his positive to give them.

It is easy to see that mind makes the nerve bundles to vibrate as that. If we are angry, it vibrates very strongly which affect the quiet vibrations around us. If we are quiet, our quiet vibrations will reassure the patient. Therefore the qigong master must be completely self-sufficient to balance with the vibrations around.

We also possible to give a privilege for qi by concentrating thought, self-suggest, gentle yet continuous on the impression he wants to make. Do not let anything distract your mind. The mind must to be quiet, persevering, not showing out with gestures like clenched hands but just a determination inside. Do you want to plant anger on the opposite person? Make this mood in your mind by focusing your thoughts. That way, thoughts affect the qi and cause the corresponding vibrations. There is no need to clench your hands, raise your fist, harden, jump or scream. Experience shows that just mental effort, mellow and continuous is that enough to directly affect the mental strength.

On the other hand, do you want to put someone in a quiet, relaxed state? Let him sit down, put his hands on his thighs, and you sit opposite, put your hands on his hands. Relax your muscles and try to express the silence and comfort which you want to convey by concentrating thought. If trained, you can create this mood easily in minutes. The more you live in that state of mind, the more you make other person feel it.

Those who know self-control will succeed in qigong, whether experiential or healing. If you cure a person with a nervous breakdown or anemia, do not react, do not decide, you should excite them. You need to visualize in your thought that the patient as energetic full, healthy enough to live normal. By concentrating your mind constantly, you will create the good mood in your mind which includes strength, volition, self-command then your qi will bring to the patient this style and make him stronger.

Conversely, when treating a patient who is angry, you must feel calm inside to transfer it to the sick person. Do not think that this is just a game of imagination, experience shows that the thought affects the qi flow, concentrates or distribute it as your wanting and give it the vibration necessary for the treatment.

To understand this, consider the following experiment by Lord William Crookes, the great scholar of England. He proved that natural agents such as sound, electricity, heat, light... are formed by different levels of vibration. He took a clock to tap each second to get started and then ascend the tap beat. At the level of 32 vibrations per second or more, sound appears: it is the lowest music note. The vibration is higher, the sound is higher. The human ear listens to the sound at level 32,768 vibrations per second. When the vibrations are raised beyond the sound level, the heat, light, and electricity appear. In this vibration scale, we think of qi. Just as the sound goes from 32 to 32,768 vibrations per second that the human ear hears, the qi must also have a wide range from the weakest vibrations to the strongest vibrations. This is the role of the will to increase or decrease these vibrations. Although there is no concrete evidence to support this hypothesis, this is also suggests clear that we can understand the effects of emotions and thoughts on qi flow.

The mind not only transmits a vibration to the qi, but it also delivers the qi outward, releasing the qi in a certain direction. Therefore, when we release the qi into someone, we must look in the middle of our forehead (the center of attention) or in the "positive plexus" (under the sternum) to focus the attention and drive the direction of the qi power. Thus, the will has a huge effect on enhancing and guiding to release the qi. The strong qigong masters do not need to be pretend, they just look at the patient with a determined mind then the subject feels the desired effect, without suggestive words or autosuggestion. The patient is often unknown before and still feels effective, sometimes far away. But to be successful first, the patient must be sensitive. The use of thought to heal is only achieved after years of practice. Before achieving that, it is better to use gestures to release the qi in a certain direction.

Chapter 4

The qi release by hand waving technique

There are two types of hands waving: vertical and horizontal. Vertical waving is the hand starting at the top of the head and waving down along the patient's body. Do not strain, do not use force; the hands are loose, the fingers are not close together, nor separated away; palms downward. Raise your hand as lightly as the air lifted. Lower your hand slowly, as if you want to use your fingers to point out five vertical lines on the body, or evenly distributed from above to a substance that we poured from the head down. When our hand is down lowest, we clench into fists to hold the qi because it continues to emit. We lift two fists up the patient's head along the two sides, without the front line as it can disturb the effect of the wave down. When we bring the fist up to the top of our head, we open our hands to pour out something - this is the specifics of the thought - which we distribute on the patient's body through the action down.

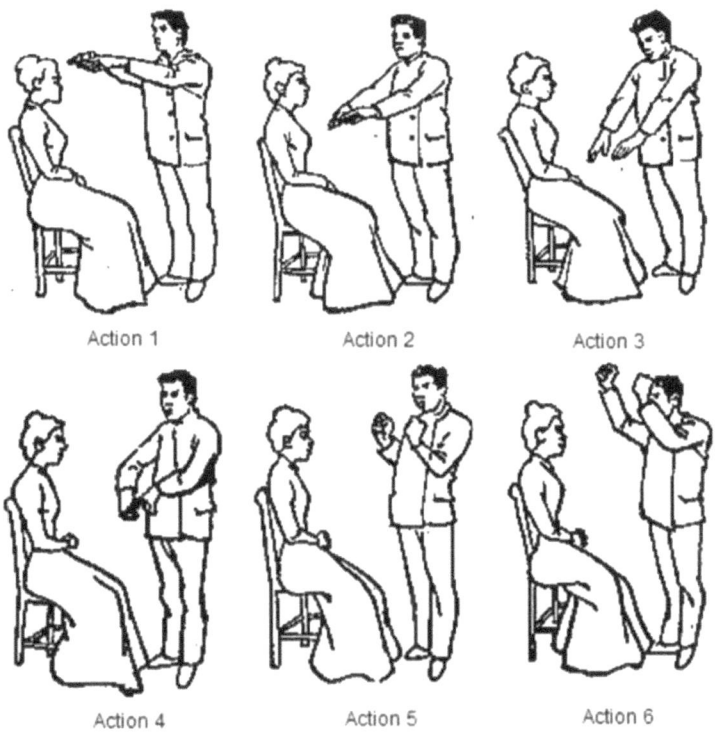

Figure 3 - The vertical waving technique

Sometimes we need hands waving from the head to the patient's feet, but sometimes we just wave from the head to their part of their body. For example, when we want to bring the patient to sleep, we waved slowly from head to upper abdomen like releasing qi, leading qi and condensation to the "positive mess". There are cases where we just waved with one hand, such as limited effects on a narrow area or an organ of the patient. We move the elliptical hand in front of the part that needs treatment, waving to the sick person's body and moving the patient away from the patient before returning to the starting point. It is important to avoid the effect of hand-waving to be disabled by hand lift. Waving down creates an qi flow inside the patient's body, so the hand lift which are too close to them will cause this effect to be disturbed or disrupted. Note that hands are only 5 to 10 cm from the patient when waving down, while lifting hands then right hand away from 30 to 40 cm. Some authors advise us to wave in the opposite direction. It is a guide that should never be followed because it has many disadvantages. Especially for those who are prone to excitement, waving from the legs to the head often causes discomfort, which can cause them to vomit.

The waving is fast or slow depending on the desired effect. Slowly waving - Each time about 30 seconds for the distance from head to belly is additional method. Waving is done with a quiet will, wanting to nourish the patient's body, want to strengthen their mental capacity. If waving is right then there is a clear qi change from the qi gong master to the patient, who will have a pleasant, relaxed feeling and feel a new a new vitality from about fifteen minutes to half an hour later. Waving faster is the method of subtracting. With this method, the will to be also quiet and want to reduce the stimulation of the patient. Patients often feel a stream of cool air inside the body follow the waving action of the physician. Of course, the qi gong master must have a strong will toward the desired outcome, accompanied by the suggestive autism and a sustained mental focus. Note: Slowly waving from the head to the abdomen causing the patient to sleep, while fast waving to wake them up.

Next is the horizontal waving. First, the arms are crossed in front of the chest and spread out horizontally; then move in the opposite direction to bring the hands back to the original position. To be more specific, in the early stages, the forearms were piled up in the middle of the chest, palms toward the patient, thumbs underneath, the other fingers spread out. Then move your arms to two sides in a spinning motion, but the palms still point towards the patient, the thumbs still below. The arms continued to extend, forearms and hands rotated. The arms are stretched horizontally, the palms still pointing towards the patient and the fingers are spread out. In the second phase, the forearms are back, while turning the hands back to their original position.

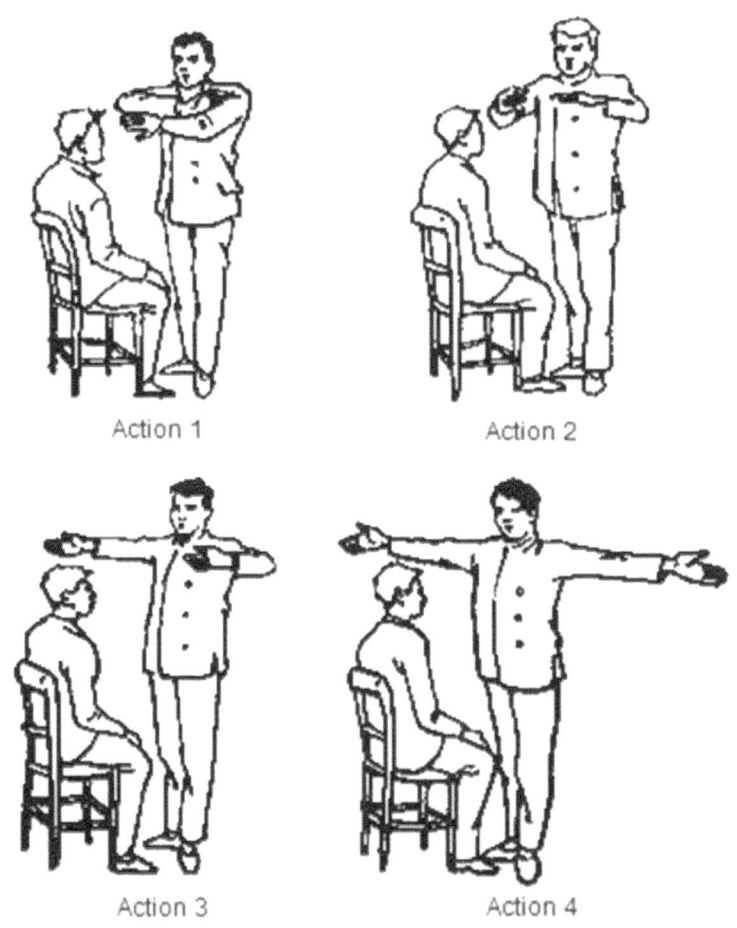

Figure 4 - The horizontal waving technique

Perform a series of hand-waving movements about 20 to 30 cm from the patient; The hands that propel the air in front of the patient, which will lead to effective subtracting and relief of the patient. This should be done in front of face or in front of the chest of patient who is depressed, weighed head or congested. The action just a few minutes is enough to bring them back to a relaxed and calm mind.

Chapter 5

The qi release technique to a point

The qi release technique to a point named "hold" which has a great importance. The qi receiving area is a certain organ or organ of the patient. To do this, the qi gong master places his or her hand or finger in front of the affected part at a certain distance. The qi release by hand is done by placing the palms 5 to 20 cm away from the treated part and holding it there for a period of 1 to 5 minutes. Usually use only one hand, but sometimes use both. Properly following the yin and yang rules, "hold" will has the additional or subtracting effectively.

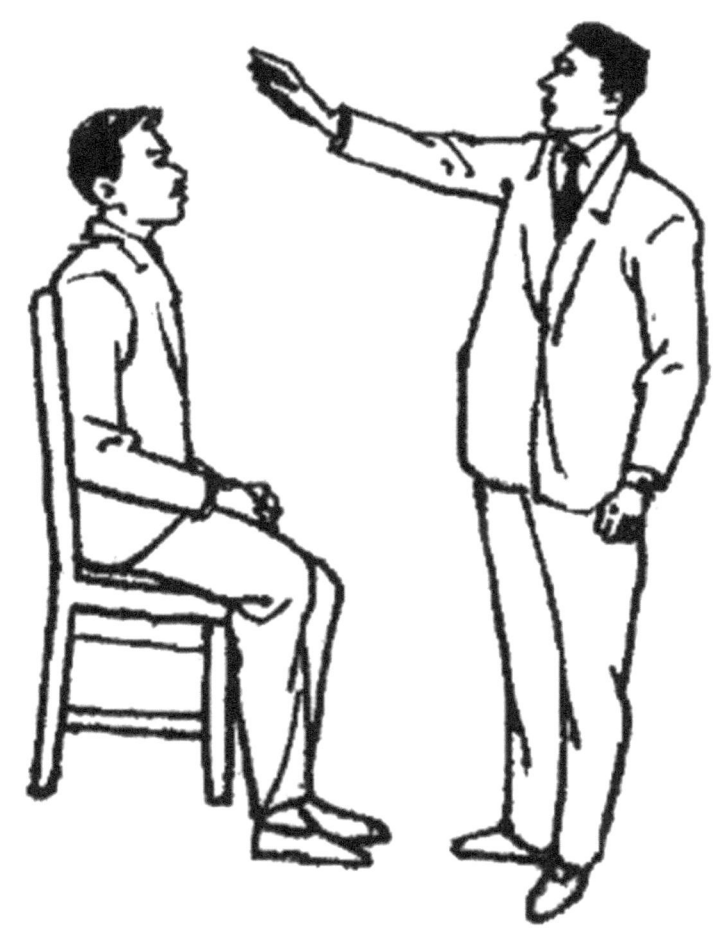

Figure 5 - The qi release by a palm

It is important to note that the qi gong master must relax the muscles. This also applies to all other tricks. Never stretch muscles. The action must be very smooth. The first reason is to save energy, because muscle tension will waste some energy without benefit to anyone. The second reason is that stiff muscles will block the flow of qi. The need for a qi gong master is self-control, no restlessness, anger or emotion.

The qi release technique by fingers is done with right hand. The fingers are straight, not touching, not moving, toward and 10 to 15 cm away from the treated part. Directly using the fingers to add or subtract depending on the wishes of the qigong master. For strong effect, the fingers bunched, drawing the circle in front of the treated part. This is the only method of qi circle release, it has stimulating effect. For example, use this method for the intestines to stimulate the contractions which treat constipation.

To further enhance the effect, attention should be paid to the yin and yang rules: the yang elements opposite together or yin facing yin then them make an extra efficiency. In contrast, yang faces yin or yin faces yang make a less effect. So, if the qigong master wants to supplement the patient then his right hand must to place in front of their chest or his left hand placed in the area behind their back. Generally, releasing qi by the right hand is greater effectiveness, except for left-handed people. Another point to keep in mind is to move the qigong master's hand in a circle from left to right - clockwise above the patient's body with the clock facing the qigong master. Do it to increase the qi for the receiver.

In addition, the other way of qi releasing is more powerful, is to launch the finger with the rotation of the hand like to drill holes. The qigong master imagines like holding a drill to drill a hole in the board. The qigong master turn his hand to the right and relax, then turn his hand to the left to turn the "drill"; Repeat until he wants to stop. This operation is done by hand without another tool, only with the fingers pointing at the part that needs treatment. Some sensitive people will feel the intestinal tightening when activated on the abdomen by this method and find it necessary to go to the toilet immediately.

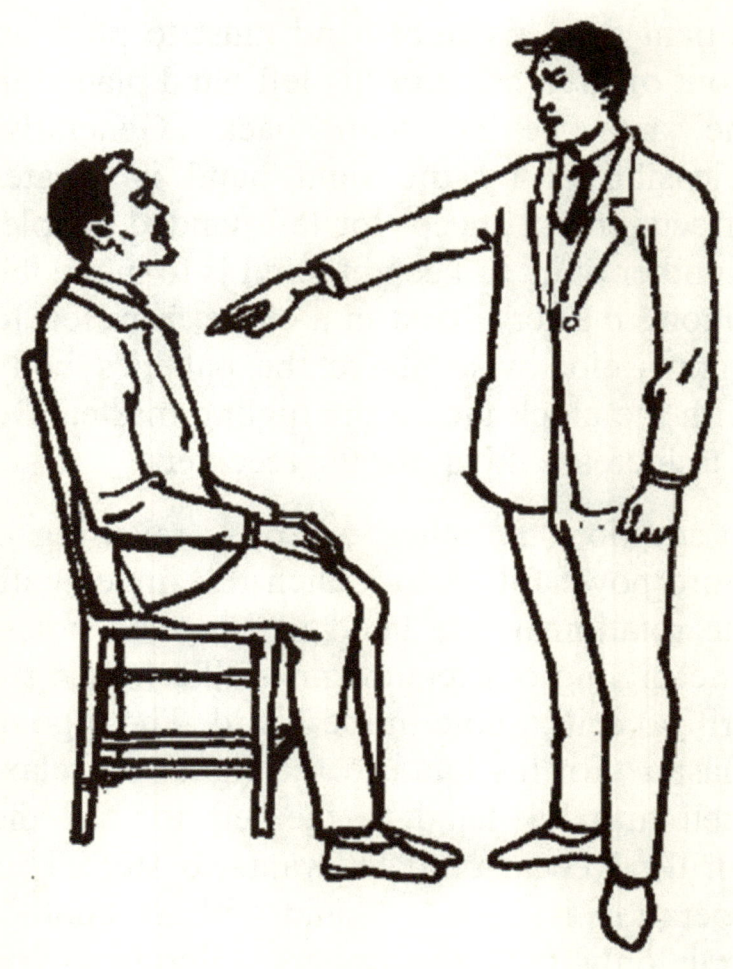

Figure 6 - The qi release by fingers

Chapter 6

The qi release by massaging techniques

The biggest difference in the method of qi releasing by massaging with the above mentioned methods is that the hands of the qi gong master touch the patient's body. There are many tricks in this method. Place a fixed hand on the treated part for a long or short time depending on the desired effect is that called "close up". For large parts such as chest, abdomen or back, should use both hands close up gently on it, do not press down. The hands are so loose to release gas smoothly and do not waste energy. When the qi gong master need to treat an organ or viscera such as the heart, eyes, stomach, or a narrow body such as the forehead or the nape, he or she uses one hand.

The "close up" method makes an additional or subtracting effects also follows the yin and yang rules which are shown at chapter 5. For example, to making "reducing effect" in the area of the forehead, heart or stomach of patient, the qi gong master needs to put the left hand on it; if he wants to have "additional effect" then he uses his right hand. For other example, the qi gong master wants to create a "reducing effect" on the patient's chest. The patient sits back in the chair, the qigong master sitting opposite, touching his right hand on patient's left chest and his left hand on right chest for a long time. If the patient need a "additional effect" on his chest area, the qigong master move to cross two hands, the left hand on the left chest and right hand on the right chest of the patient.

Caress is the second trick which is a common method for massage and qigong. The only difference is that when the massage is stroked on the skin and the doctor's hand touching the skin of the patient, while the qigong is action outside their clothes. Clothing is not a barrier and it is also a qi permeable material, which can bring qi into the body gradually. The qigong master gently caress on the part that needs treatment, with the hands smoothed, the muscles are not strained. Caressing actions are performed on all parts of the body, from top to bottom or in circles as in the abdomen. Another point to note is that in massage, physicians often recommend stroking from the outside inward, in the direction to inside. In contrast, in qigong, in order to have effect on the nervous and blood circulation, stroking from top to bottom, from head to foot in the direction to outside.

Caress has the effect of reducing, reassuring, soothe. Want to caress the body, starting from the top to the abdomen, then caress from the chest to the hands. Patient sitting, physician standing opposite, stroking with two hands, through two stages: First, the qigong master place his hands on the sides of patient's head, thumbs pointing straight at the center of the head, 3 to 4 cm apart; The other fingers slightly out, on the ears. The hand slightly curled, clawed across the ear, both sides of the neck, shoulders forearm to the tip of the finger. Next, the qigong master takes his hands back to the original position and caress down patient's neck, chest to patient's abdomen. Repeat this way about 5, 6 times, then the qigong master sits down in front of the patient, put his hands to the chest and caress down the stomach, intestines, thighs, and legs, then stroke from chest to hip, through liver, kidneys and the outside of the legs. Patients may lie in the same way as the above.

Addition, the qigong master also can be swept on the back spine: patient sitting back straight, the qigong master's hand between back and seat; he stands to the left of the patient, his left hand placed on patient's forehead or chest, gently moves it with his right arm down from patient's nape to waist. When swiping to the bottom of the spine, remember to take your hand away before moving up slowly to continue like that but not counteract the effect of the swiping down.

To treat a part, such as the stomach or intestines, the patient can sit or lie and relax his muscles while the qigong master sits or stands on the right to use his right hand. The stomach lies just below the ribs, containing food with the exit on the right. So it is necessary to swing from the left to the right, in a half-circle at the navel with the protrusions above for promoting the work of the stomach and the movement of food in it. When the intestine is lazy, stroke from the bottom of the pelvic bone to the right, around the navel, to the bottom left to return to the original position, continue to stroke the circle. Strongly caress has enhanced stimulation; slow to get the effect of reduce, soothe and relieve abdominal pain.

Next, strong caress is called "rub". When you caress, your hands lightly move on the skin. When you rub, your hands squeeze down by muscles. There are two types of straightening and circles rubbing. The straight rubbing is done slowly, from top to bottom, along the communication system and muscles of body. The fingers are spread out and slightly curved so that the entire hand is in contact with the patient's body. When you do the rubbing, you have to mobilize the joints, with a series of downward movements, like pushing and pulling something on the skin of the person. The straight rubbing is stimulating. Rubbing along the ribs, along the path of muscular and intercostal nerves, will quickly dissipate any stagnation or shortness of breath. The diseases prescribed for this procedure are shortness of breath, asthma or fatigue, headache. Patient sitting relaxed, loose muscles; the qigong master standing or sitting opposite, hands under the patient's arm behind his back. Rubbing from the spine to the front of the chest, try to follow the ribs, fingers placed on the rib slits to affect the intercostal muscles, increase their mobility and help to breathe easy. Just a few minutes are enough. The circle rubbing is to put the hand near the part that needs treatment such as intestines, heart, liver, kidneys ... and rub the circle on it. The circle rubbing also has the effect of stimulating to the affected parts. The rubbing movements must be clockwise (the clock on the patient with the watch face toward the physician) to stimulate and transfer the qi from the qigong master to the patient.

Chapter 7

The qi release by blowing techniques

The blowing of the qigong master has effect of strong qi releasing. From ancient times, it was the image of the transfer of life force. Theologians claim that God gave the soul man with his breath that makes people different from other animals. It was the same blow that the qigong master treated the disease miraculously. Anyway, we must also say that blowing is a very powerful, effective application to healing. There are two types of blowing: warm blowing is yang and cold blowing is yin. Warm blowing is performed on the patient's body or slightly away. The qigong master opens his mouth and slowly, long blows the air which has accumulated in the lungs. It is possible to blow a distance of 1 or 2 cm, but it is better to blow close to the patient's skin on a suction object such as cloth, felt or cotton wool. Place the mouth on this object and blow to in it, then inhale deeply to continue. Stronger blows will produce the corresponding effect. Blowing on the chest will restore the heartbeat to stop the fainting within 2 or 3 blows. Practice deep breaths, the longer and stronger blowing. Warm blowing can save patients in situations of despair. That is transfer of true vitality. Contraindicated is in cases of severe heart or blood vessel disease and severe pulmonary tuberculosis, because the patient's body cannot withstand a strong reaction.

"Cold blowing" is always done remotely. The qigong master pursed lips as if to blow out the candles. This blowing style has soothing effect.

Not just the blow of the qigong master, but his eyes can also transmit qi to heal. The effect of the eyes is strong or weak depending on the intensity of the look and the time of attentiveness. The first thing to notice is that hypnosis should not be used, as it makes the patient feel very tired and bloody in the eye, leading to a variety of discomfort such as blindness, heat, prickles in the eyes and headache. Remove all aggression, which can cause the patient's body to resist and not produce the desired effect. Only the new mellow methods are not harmful to the physiological and psychological balance of the patient. Hypnosis is made very close (the nose of the physician near the nose of the patient) causing the patient's eye to be deviated and the person who suffering from neurological disease can suffer a dangerous seizure.

Thus, the look of the qigong master must be firm, assertive but attentive mellow. The qigong master do not roll his eyes, it may seem ridiculous to make the patient laugh and harmful to the effect of treatment. Look straight in the middle of the forehead, above the intersection of two eyebrows, the center of attention. In addition to the effect on the patient, this view is very good for the qigong master to avoid any mental dispersion. If patient need to soothe then the thought of the qigong master must be mellow. If patient need to excitement then the qigong master must focus on the qi flow. The qigong master looks at the patient from a distance of 2 to 3 meters, causing a long-lasting relaxation which is very good for patients with acute illness, discomfort, anger and excitability.

If the patient lie, the qigong master stands at the end of the bed or next to the foot of the patient, looking at the intersection of two eyebrows or "positive mess", with a calm will, feeling completely relax, the soothing sensation of the body. The look will bring the feeling of relaxation to the patient. The qigong master takes more stable-self, the higher efficiency. Patients upset, rolling back and forth will quiet for between 15 minutes to half an hour and can sleep peacefully.

Chapter 8

The objects hold qi

Some of the objects that attract and hold qi can be used as capacitors to put the desired effect into the body. Qigong therapy uses this type of indirect qi transfer. Between the two sessions, the qigong master can place the cloth or gauze (which contained qi) over the patient's pain area to bring the qi into the body continuously and intensively.

The qi is brought into the body by food directly affects the function of the digestive system. From there it has been remarkably successful in healing, not only in the stomach and intestines, but also in the liver, spleen, kidney and bladder. This is usually prescribed in chronic diseases such as constipation persistent, stomach loss of ability to contract, jaundice, malaria… The patients are on the diet of vegetables and water or medications which were exposed to qi. These foods and drinks greatly affect organ function, rebalance and promote excretion. Not all things hold the same qi. There is more or less qi suction according to each type. The liquid, especially water, the most qi holding, drink half a glass of qi containing water when hungry will cure the disease of the digestive system. Fabrics, wool, felt and cotton wool are also good qi attractants. In addition, ancient qigong master used fats such as oils, waxes, moisturizing cream... to absorb qi. All of these materials are used to provide continuous qi to the next treatment. When it is not possible to directly treat it, the qigong master can transfer qi to these objects to place on the pain part and the results are also very positive. The metal also absorbs gas, but needs to distinguish yin and yang characteristics, such as iron is yang and copper is yin.

Want to impregnate qi on a certain object, hold it in the palm for several minutes, "waving" or "pointing" on it and blowing in it if needed. In about 10 minutes, the object has absorbed enough qi.

In order to transfer qi into a water bottle, place it on a high table, avoiding the metal as it makes qi escape. Hands hold the water bottle for 5 or 10 minutes, waving along the bottle height, and "pointing" on the mouth of bottle, with the right hand with the fingers bunched up, while the left hand holds the bottle. If the water in it is used outside, blow into the mouth of bottle. Fifteen minutes or half an hour is enough to infuse qi of one liter of water. If the water in another object should choose a round object such as brass pot or cup because the qi tends to escape at the sharp angles. Notice the yin and yang rules: impregnate yang qi with your right hand and slightly warm blowing, impregnate yin qi with your left hand and cold blowing.

Do the following: release qi in two glasses of water, one with the right hand, one with the left hand and do not let the patient know. Ask the patient to drink each glasses of water and ask them to talk about their feelings. If the patient is sensitive, they will find that the yang water is easily absorbed, and the yin water is bland, uncomfortable and nauseous.

The qi is not only in humans but also in animals and minerals. Man is not the only one who can emit the yin qi and yang qi, all things in nature can do the same. However, the thing is that in the qi flow which plants release has the effect makes sleepy. The superficial observers thought that the scent of plants was the cause of this effect, but many plants without incense also emit qi.

Dr. Chaprignon experimented with the following: he placed on the medicinal plant the surface of the treated part, and then release qi to bring the medicinal effect to the inside body for producing the desired effect. For example: to relieve the pain of malignancy, he put the opium on the part of the pain, then release qi, resulting in quiet patients and sleep like eating opium.

Dr. Bouryu and Burot of Rochefort Medical School tried to place the opium on the patient's head. The medicine is wrapped in paper to avoid any suggestion-self. About a minute later, the patient's eyelids collapse, muscles soften, head rests on the pillow, breathing harmonic. Ten minutes later, the patient awakened, yawned, rubbed his eyes and is alert as after normal sleeping. Then, the opium was put on the patient's nape, forehead, hands, soles of the feet, the result always the same.

However, not everyone is affected by the drug when it is near. If so, the pharmacy staff will quit. Only sensitive people will recognize such small qi rays. To ordinary people, it is the qi release of qigong master that helps them absorb the effect of the drug to inside. And do not forget that the results do not have to be immediately, they need a certain amount of time.

Chapter 9

Healing by qigong

The body is healthy when organs work well, but there are many causes that disrupt human functions. First of all, agencies can only work in its limited capacity. If this limit is exceeded, the organs will suffer wear and be damaged quickly. When we force the stomach to work too hard to digest too much food, it loses elasticity. Overeating not only disables the stomach but also damages the liver and kidneys overwork. The heart is a pump that draws red blood to the lungs to clean up and then delivers this clean blood throughout the body. The heart works so hard by a lot of the cause as sadness, anxiety, night, excessive pleasure. If the heart works too much red blood will not return to the heart quickly and stagnant along the way cause headache, difficulty breathing, nosebleeds, varicose veins, treatment, menstruation more. In addition, the blood does not carry enough oxygen, causing toxicity disturbing other organs. In order to compensate for this, the heart will increase the pulse, so that the nervousness and complications are severe.

The cause of the body's imbalance is a lot, but roughly can be said is that because of not respect the natural law made the disease appear. Most dysfunction can be avoided if we only provide enough food for the body, do not clog it and do not force it over work. Those who follow the normal rules are physically and emotionally well-both involved - and happy. Living like that also prevents the bacteria that cause the disease. This may not sound right to some people, but it has been proven, if it is not all of the bacteria then at least in large numbers. Patients with tuberculosis or cancer are comforted and encouraged to effectively fight bacterial invasions and prolong their lives, although their weakened body is prone to disease. This is the problem of self healing. We all have "Koch" bacteria but not everyone has tuberculosis. Only weak people do nothing to fight the new disease. We can treat all illnesses ourselves or at least delay the progression of serious illnesses.

In nature, there are two elements that are inseparable from matter and energy. We find both in the human body. The material makes up the skeleton and the body, energy makes the organs operate. As such, health issues are retracted in the following two proposals: The first, create a good body that is resistant to disease by providing food reasonably. The second maintain a balance of energies.

Illness is the loss of balance of energies. Want to heal, just restore that balance. Remember that medication can't make balancing because it does not work on the whole body. Drug affects only one organ, always detrimental to another. Pain relievers are harmful to the stomach. The medication cures swollen joints to damage kidney. Medicine uses drugs to treat symptoms that do not address the cause of the disease, so it does not heal. For example, opium only relieves pain and does not treat the wound. This is the limit of modern medicine. There is only one means of healing, that is, the balance of all the energies in the body. The meaning of "body synchronization system" should be the main part of all cures. Paddy rice cannot be planted in dry fields like the disease cannot develop on a healthy body. Therefore, a body with a good immune system can fight against millions of germs in it. We all have many inflammatory causes, but only the weak persons are ill. I can say about hundreds of such cases.

If effective healing only is limited to the problem of "self-balancing system", then cure will be very simple. Yes, good cure is very simple. Is simplicity a characteristic of great truths? The more advanced the invention, the simpler it becomes. A new technology requires up to ten sets of machines that only need one later. An artwork that wants to be beautiful and true must be simple. Medical therapy should be as simple as that.

The first thing that a physician must do is tell the patient the cause of the disease and convince him of the need to live as close to nature as possible. Help the patient to resist the illness by "suggesting" and gain new energy by qigong. The "suggestion" effects on psychology, qigong effects on physiology. In the first method, the very thought that decides the healing, in the second method, it is the "transfer of force". Two different methods, but they complement each other.

The qi does not have medicine properties but only make balances. The qi's impact is more pronounced when the body's balance is broken. The more physically or mentally impaired the patient, the more sensitivity to qigong. This sensitivity decreases as the patient recovers. Patients will know when to stop treatment. Emphasize again the role of qi in healing. In case of emergency, we can use hot blowing air to let a weak body taking an outburst of vitality. At the threshold of death, the patient can also find his health.

For effective treatment, only the patient puts him-self or her-self in calm state of physically and emotionally, letting relax his muscles and follow the healing. Patients do not need to be convinced about the effect of qigong to treat the disease. Qigong is an independent agent for any suggestion or suggestive self. When treated with qigong, some people do not feel anything. However, the effect of qigong on the physiology of the patient is real. There are people who feel very clearly in front of the qigong master's hands like shivering, warm, cool, yawning, heavy head, sleepy.

Deep research on restoring balance of the body, illness is a consequence of the loss of balance as mentioned above. Balances go away in two ways: the body parts work above or below the average. Over the average, excessively active organs can lead to inflammation. Under average, the body's functioning decreases, slows down, can progress to paralysis. This division is very simple, but it helps us understand the basic principle of treatment by qigong. For example, stomach overwork, contraction faster, producing more fluid, leading to cramping, stiff neck, hunger, stomach pain or stomach inflammation. In contrast, if the stomach is weak, the loss of tonic, discomfort, poor eating, digestion difficult. Of course, in case the head must be subtracted, the following case must be added. The guiding principle of qigong healing is to add energy to the weakened organs and to diminish energy of the too strong organs. However, in some chronic diseases such as rheumatism, gout... there are occasional severe pain, it is better to "subtracting" the pain and "additional" the whole body, especially the organs digestion and excretion. Patients relieve the stagnation substances, the joints will recover as soon as possible.

The contents that presented in the previous sections may give general ideas of how to treat ills by qigong. Carefully memorize the yin and yang of the body, we will create additional or subtracting effects easily (see Figures 7).

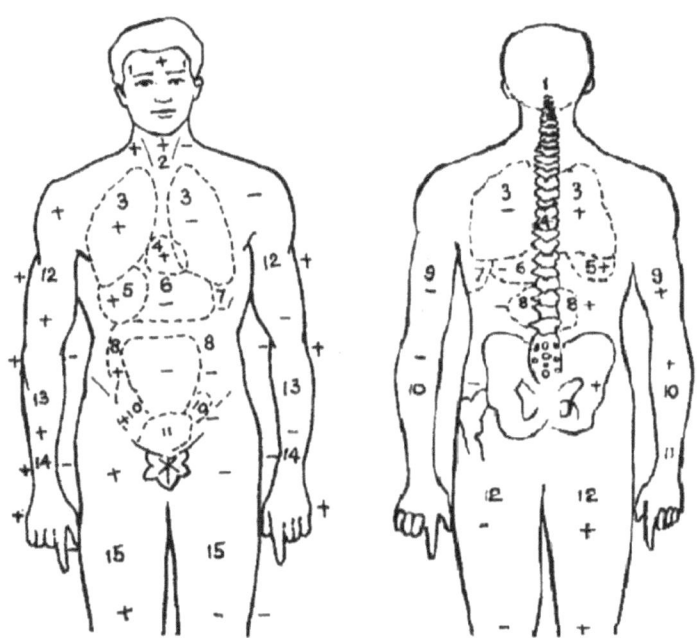

Figure 7 - The yin and yang divisions of the body

Also, it is necessary to repeat as follows: the two opposite polarities touch together to "subtract" (+ with - or - with +), the same polarities touch together to "addition" (+ with + or - with -). From these instructions, we can deduce how to behave in different situations.

Note: Before treatment, the qigong master needs to create the balance relationship between him with the patient's body and bring the patient into a state of mental and physical tranquility. To do that, the patient need to sit comfortably, his limbs relaxed, his hands on his lap (not crossed his arms), his back resting on the chair, not reluctant to the thinking of healing. The qigong master sits in front of the patient, his hand on the patient's hand, the thumb of the two persons touching each other, his knees and feet closely together for 10 or 15 minutes. Each treatment begins with this relationship, but gradually decreases down time. Next, start doing the tricks of "addition" or "subtract".

For example of headache treatment, the qigong master will stand to the left of the patient, place the left hand (-) on the forehead (+) and the right hand (+) on the patient's neck (-). After 10 or 20 minutes, he will massage the patient's spine with his right hand. In contrast, treatment of head's ischemia, the qigong master needs to supplement. He stands on the right of the patient, the right hand (+) on the forehead (+), the left hand (-) on the back (-).

At the end of the treatment, relax the patient by "horizontal waving" and "vertical waving" throughout the length of the body, then blowing to the patient's head and chest.

The will of qigong master has a great influence on qi release. So he needs to take advantage of the will. He must create in his spirit the style that he wants to impose on the sick. His self-control, maturity, and morale are very important factors.

Chapter 10

Practice qigong to healing

In order to have enough vigor to heal, you have to charge the qi every day and recharge the qi after the treatment. To release qi, we must know the way of qi condensing, then the drive qi to the tip of the finger to then release to other people. This is an elaborate practice that requires years of practice, cannot be fully described in a book chapter.

Below is a summary of the qigong exercise process that can be used to treat the disease:

First, condense qi to a certain place in the body. Men usually use their low belly which is away from the bottom of the navel a hand. Women use the upper abdomen which is the indentation between the breasts. The yogis use the "positive plexus" at the bottom of the breastbone. The evidence of qi condensing in one part of your body is warm, pleasant, gradually warming up to the point where it wants to move to other parts of your body.

Next, use the "mind" to leads the warm qi follow the spine to the top of the head, through three narrow places called "three doors". Taoist calls this "sub heaven circle", yoga called "fire snake" (Kundalini shakti).

When the two front and back channels are smooth, we use the idea to bring that warm qi from the spine to the limbs. This is the "great heaven circle" of the Tao. Tai Chi provides the most perfect exercises.

Finally, practice to shoot out the qi to turn off the candle. Finished elaborately, just continue to practice every day for further development.

Important note: The necessary condition for qi recharge is physical and mental relaxation. You have to forget your little human and only see the vast universe, then the new energy is full, never exhausted.

After the end of treatment for patients, you lie on your back, let loose muscular body, deep breathing, light and regular. Your mind is focused on the atmosphere, in harmony with the universe then your body will recharge enough the qi to supplement the loss. This is the "Savasana" posture of yoga.

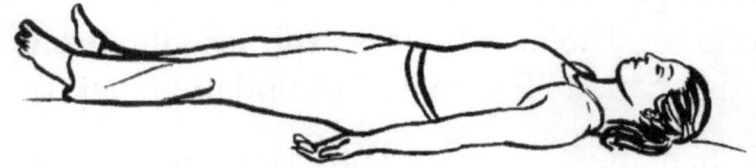

Figure 8 - The posture of qi recharging

Conclusions

The therapeutic method of qi has existed since ancient times, everywhere there are, although they are called under different names such as treatment by human's bioelectric or vibrated field. If this method were "miracles" in the past, only a handful of people could do it, now in the light of science, through scientific experimentation, its superstition has vanished gradually. People have seen the qi, photographed it, measured its rays with modern machinery and learned its effects in many different fields. The qigong masters of India or China today have demonstrated that qigong in general and therapeutic qigong in particular are scientific in nature that anyone can practice as long as they have proper instruction by the masters. The contents of this book do not make you the qigong master immediately, but it is very important for those who are interested in qi using to care health. Principles of disease cause that mentioned in chapter 9 are very simple to help the people have the right explanation and healthy lifestyle to prevent illness. The techniques of qigong masters are described in detail in the chapter 4, chapter 5, chapter 6 and chapter 7 to help the reader visualize the whole picture of the qi healing. Also, the yin and yang divisions of the human body that mentioned in the chapter 2 and chapter 9 is the most fundamental knowledge. All are the new and important to the newbie in this field. They also help build our confidence in health care and treatment based on ancient elite intellectual knowledge. Finally, we end this book with a quote from the healing yoga book by Dr. Phulgenda Sinha as follows: "Each individual must be responsible for the cause of his or her own illness as well as treatment".

The end

The books were published by the author

01- Feng Shui for Beginners

02- View by Qi

03- Applications of the Yin-Yang and Bagua

04- 12 Chinese Zodiac Signs - For Self Discovery and Team Building

05- The Wondrous Strategies of Ancient China (Outside of 36 Tricks)

06- Feng Shui For East Facing Houses - In Period 8 (2004 - 2023)

07- Feng Shui For West Facing Houses - In Period 8 (2004 - 2023)

08- Feng Shui For South Facing Houses - In Period 8 (2004 - 2023)

09- Feng Shui For North Facing Houses - In Period 8 (2004 - 2023)

10- Feng Shui For South East Facing Houses - In Period 8 (2004 - 2023)

11- Feng Shui For North West Facing Houses - In Period 8 (2004 - 2023)

12- Secrets to Success - Colors of Feng Shui 2018

13- Secrets to Success - Colors of Feng Shui 2017

14- Feng Shui for 2018

15- Feng Shui for 2017

16- Feng Shui For 2016

Visit to purchase these books to continue reading more. Show the author you appreciate their work!